"For cardiac arrest, simply calling 9-1-1 won't work, the EMT's or Paramedics will arrive too late with their defibrillator, and the patient will usually die. There is a better way..."

— Lance Hodge, Paramedic

An AED at HOME:
A New Paradigm for Saving Lives

ISBN-13: 978-1986187183

Printed in the United States of America

Updated: 9/2020

An AED at HOME:
A New Paradigm for Saving Lives

By Lance Hodge

Paradigm: *a model, pattern, a norm.*

Paradigm shift: *a profound change in a fundamental model*

~

"We need a new paradigm for saving lives from cardiac arrest. What we've been doing for 50 years isn't working. We can save tens of thousands of lives every year, if we just make some simple changes."

-Lance Hodge, Paramedic

Forward...

Family and bystanders often don't know what to do in a life-threatening medical emergency. 9-1-1 help from EMT's and Paramedics often arrives too late and people die that might have been saved.

I'm a Paramedic, I've been a Paramedic since 1980 and worked in a big city fire department. Now I teach a college EMT course. I've written some simple guidebooks on the basics of CPR and First Aid, but without expensive marketing few will read them.

Too often the people at the scene of a medical emergency have no idea what to do, they simply call 9-1-1 and think that that is enough. *Sometimes* that is enough. But in the case of a *respiratory arrest* (someone who has a pulse but is not breathing) or a *cardiac arrest* (no pulse and no breathing) calling 9-1-1 *isn't* enough; EMT's and Paramedics will often arrive too late to save these people!

Particularly with *cardiac arrest*, the help the victim needs MUST reach them **in the first few minutes** or their brain will suffer irreversible damage, and most likely they will die. The help they need is the *defibrillator*. A simple defibrillator that requires almost no training is the AED. The *Automated External Defibrillator.*

Modern Emergency Medical Services began about fifty years ago. For cardiac arrest, it's not working. This book is about *saving tens of thousands of lives* by changing our approach to cardiac arrest and thinking in new and innovative ways.

Lance Hodge

Chapter One

We can do better. 50 years of prehospital Emergency Medicine, EMT's and Paramedics, improved 9-1-1 dispatch systems and training, and millions, if not billions of dollars invested to save more people in cardiac arrest, and... it's not working. Now what?

I'll repeat the punchline right here, the treatment that saves people in cardiac arrest is **defibrillation**.
A simple to use defibrillator, the **AED** (Automated External Defibrillator) is on ambulances and firetrucks and is often available in many public buildings and businesses. If a cardiac arrest occurs when a defibrillator is close by, the person might live.

Most cardiac arrests occur at **home**, about **80%** of them do, and simply calling 9-1-1 to get the defibrillator to treat the patient in cardiac arrest won't work, the EMT's or Paramedics <u>will arrive too late</u> with their defibrillator, and the patient will usually die.

There is a better way...

What we're doing doesn't work

*It's been about fifty years since "modern" EMS began. The Emergency Medical Services (EMS) is all about saving lives. Paramedics were created to save the lives of people in **Cardiac Arrest**. All those years ago, before modern EMS, we were saving about **5%** of those people in cardiac arrest.*

*Cardiac arrest means the heart has stopped beating, and when that occurs breathing also stops, and no heart beat or breathing is called DEAD. Under the right circumstances cardiac arrest may be reversed; CPR helps but it takes more. Fifty years ago, doctors in emergency rooms were frustrated that the patients arriving in cardiac arrest received their potential life-saving interventions too late, and they began to push for fire departments and ambulances to receive the advanced training and equipment that might save those lives, by getting that hospital treatment to the victims sooner, and **Paramedics** were created.*

Beginning in the late 1960's Paramedics were trained and equipped with the same equipment available in the hospital emergency room; a defibrillator, advanced airways such as endotracheal tubes, EKG monitors, and more than a dozen medications to help stabilize a cardiac rhythm after defibrillation.

*CPR has been around since the 60's and has been updated many times since. Pushing on the chest to circulate blood to the brain is nice, and helpful, but <u>CPR alone won't save these lives</u>, we must get a **defibrillator** to the patient quickly!*

The defibrillator stops the quivering of the heart (Ventricular fibrillation) that most often occurs in cardiac arrest, allowing the heart the chance to regain a functional heartbeat. Sometimes, these people in cardiac arrest can be revived, but several things must happen for them to have a chance at such resuscitation. Mostly, the defibrillator must reach them quickly!

Now, all these years later, after many millions of dollars in equipment and training, Paramedics are the norm. They were created to combat that dismal 5% save rate of people in cardiac arrest, and now, nearly 50 years later, the save rate in the United States for people in cardiac arrest is… still about 5%. We've failed.

*CPR is **one** factor that can help, but most people don't know how to do it, and if it's not done properly it's not very effective. CPR helps to keep the brain alive, by artificially pumping blood with compressions to the chest. <u>The brain will die in about 4 to 6 minutes without a proper blood supply</u>. CPR **alone** won't save the person's life, CPR buys some time, so that the brain may still be viable when the EMT's or Paramedics arrive with their defibrillator.*

The defibrillator is THE key. *<u>For every minute that goes by the chance that the defibrillator will work to reverse the cardiac arrest goes down by 10%</u>. It is common for EMS to take about 8 minutes to arrive, meaning there is an 80% chance the defibrillator will NOT work to reverse the cardiac arrest. The defibrillator must be used in the **first few minutes** to be most effective. Slightly faster response times or other fixes to the EMS system can **never** fix that basic flaw in the treatment of cardiac arrest, calling*

9-1-1 alone won't work, the EMT's and Paramedics will arrive too late with their defibrillator!

*The problem has been obvious for decades, EMT's and Paramedics don't get there in time for cardiac arrest, they CAN'T get there in time; the defibrillator must arrive at the patient's side and defibrillation must occur quickly, in the first **few** minutes following a cardiac arrest, or the person will most likely die.*

EMT's, Paramedics, Nurses and Doctors know what the problem is, but we're stuck in a failed paradigm of how things have been done in the past, and too few people are thinking outside that box. It's time we do…

Chapter Two

The New Paradigm;
Home builders as
life-savers

What can we do?

How about this…

What if home builders in the United States began putting an AED into every home they built?

The cost would be about $1,000 per new home, maybe a bit more if a fancier AED were used, less if the most basic models were used. That wouldn't affect the price of a mortgage payment, it's not a big deal for the home builder, and it's easy to do.

They could put them in a common area, I'd suggest the washer/dryer area. They already build cabinets there!

The media would be interested, and supportive, it would be big news; it's a life-saving change, it's a win-win for everyone as homebuilders would take on a whole new life-saving mission. The publicity for the home builder would be wonderful!

Other homebuilders would likely join in, and before long we would have **a new paradigm of saving lives from cardiac arrest, one spear-headed by corporations that build houses!**

It is estimated that increasing our "save" rates from cardiac arrest to just 20% would **save from 50,000 to 100,000 lives every year!**

~

Here are ten of the biggest home builders in the United States:

According to "hunker.com"

D.R. Horton

D.R. Horton is one of the leading homebuilders in the United States. Cited by Builder Magazine as America's biggest homebuilder, D.R. Horton provides homes in 28 states. With experience in providing homes since 1978, D.R. Horton emphasizes quality and value, livable floor plans and energy-efficient systems.

Pulte Homes

Pulte offers homes in 27 states in the nation, with an emphasis on innovative features, green technologies and neighborhood amenities. The Pulte Group also includes DiVosta and Del Webb, as well as their recent purchase of Centex Homes.

Lennar

Lennar Corporation, headquartered in Miami, Florida, has building projects in 17 states, according to Lennar. The company specializes in "affordable, move-up and retirement homes" for the changing needs of American families, with a focus on quality and customer service.

NVR

NVR builds homes in 25 metropolitan areas in 14 states. It was founded in 1948 during the post-war economic boom. Today, it provides homes for a wide range of demographic needs, including single-family homes, townhomes and condominiums.

KB Homes

KB Homes provides residences in 12 states in the country. With its focus on energy-efficient appliances, water-conserving systems and use of sustainable materials, KB Homes offers features and an attitude that many modern home-buyers require. KB Homes was founded in 1957.

Centex

Centex Homes, now owned by Pulte Group, offers residences in 22 states and the District of Columbia. The company was founded in 1950, and their long experience and quality are the result of keeping an eye on changing consumer needs, as well as intensive follow-up attention to its customers' feedback.

Hovnanian

K. Hovnanian Homes have provided homebuyers with quality homes since 1959. Today, Hovnanian builds houses in 17 states, with choices like retirement resort communities, high-rise condominiums, single-family homes, garden homes and estate homes.

Habitat For Humanity

Habitat for Humanity has become one of the nation's top ten homebuilders, according to the Wall Street Journal on December 21, 2010. Cutbacks from major homebuilding companies gave Habitat for Humanity's continuing record of affordable homebuilding and home rehabilitation an advantage in the current economic climate. Habitat was founded in 1976 in Americus, Georgia, as a Christian group providing housing for the disadvantaged.

The Ryland Group

Ryland Homes have provided new homes for American home-buyers since 1967. Ryland's care for both indoor and outdoor environmental quality as well as livable floorplans and careful neighborhood planning make them a favorite among American homeowners.

Beazer

Beazer Homes, headquartered in Atlanta, offers high-performance "eSmart" homes covering many price ranges and designs to appeal to American families. Beazer Homes USA, Inc. was founded in 1985.

*Those home builders, with their names in bold, are the **key** here. They are large companies with tremendous resources, talent, and influence, they build thousands and thousands of homes, and they can do something that perhaps **only** they can do; save thousands of lives of victims of cardiac arrest.*

To those home builders: *<u>Start putting AED's into the new homes you build</u>. Just that. I've written to these ten companies, asking for their support of this plan. I've sent them this book, with the promise of adding their name to Chapter Six, **"The Pioneers of Life-Saving Home Building."** Which one of those companies will be the **first**, and take the lead?*

When I update Chapter Six, I'll list the homebuilders who join this effort. I'll put out a press release about what we're doing and the companies who are leading the way. On the next page is the letter I sent to those home builders...

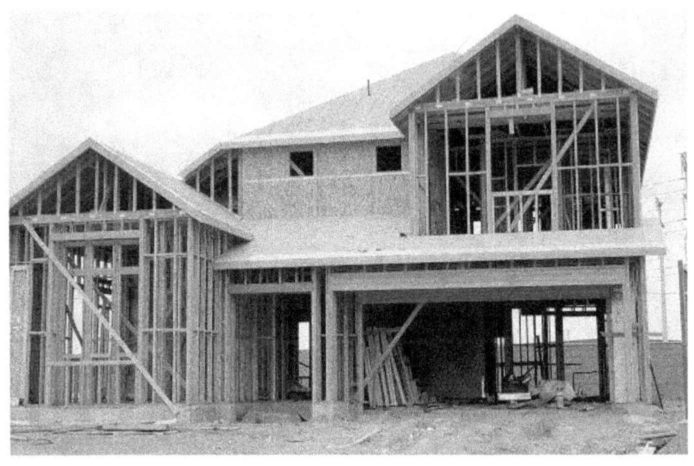

Dear Homebuilder;

I need your help.

A simple and inexpensive change can save tens of thousands of lives every year!

My name is Lance Hodge, I'm a licensed paramedic, and I've been teaching a college EMT course for more than 25 years. I worked as a *Los.Angeles City Fire Department* Paramedic for more than a decade and have responded to more than 15,000 9-1-1 calls. I know how we can save many thousands of lives every year! As a homebuilder, you can join me in this mission, and *you* can save thousands of lives.

<u>I'd like your help and involvement in getting AED/Dcfibrillators placed in new homes being built.</u> **About 350,000 people die each year from cardiac arrest.** *Nearly 80% of those cardiac arrests occur at **home**.* The *American Heart Association*® estimates that raising our "save rates" from cardiac arrest from the current 5% to 20% would save *50,000 to 100,000 lives every year!* Joining me as a partner in this effort and developing plans to put AED's in your new homes would save thousands of lives every year.

I'm not asking for any money, but I do need your help. As a major home builder, you are in a *unique* position to change the dismal survival statistics from cardiac arrest. *Saving these lives is not possible without you!*

I want to partner with you to help get AED's placed in new homes being constructed. That's all I ask, a commitment from you to begin this effort. Of course, this would be a great opportunity for positive media exposure for your company in this life-saving effort, but more importantly, those who build homes could now be the new catalyst to save lives from cardiac arrest.

I believe that the washer/dryer area should become the standard for the location of the home AED. We never know if a visitor to the home may be the one who needs to access the AED, and a standard area for placement, and a simple sign on a cabinet door, would let *everyone* always know where the AED is.

I've written a similar letter to *nine other major home builders*, and I know that *some* builder(s) will join this effort. **Someone will be the *first* and will take the lead in this effort. *You* could be that company.**

I've included a book I wrote, ***An AED at HOME: A New Paradigm for Saving Lives*** which outlines this effort. I'll update this book frequently, and in *Chapter Six* of this book I'll list the homebuilder who was ***first*** to begin this effort and others as they join.

I'll initiate a major media campaign to let the public know about this effort. With your help, we can finally and effectively begin to address those *80% of cardiac arrests that occur at **home**,* giving *thousands* of people a better chance of survival in the event of a cardiac arrest.

I would love to meet or speak with you regarding this effort, and to answer any questions you may have.

Sincerely,

Lance Hodge

Lance Hodge, Paramedic

Chapter Three

Using an AED *and* First Aid

The AED is a simple *defibrillator*. Most functions of an AED are done automatically. An AED usually has *two* buttons, one to turn it on, and one to deliver the shock to the person in cardiac arrest.

Anyone is allowed to use an AED if there is one available. *Good Samaritan laws* in virtually every state protect you from liability if you act responsibly in your efforts to help during a medical emergency.

Note:
*Some AED's will also guide you on how to perform proper CPR, some will only provide a shock, and won't help you to do CPR. The "**Zoll AED-Plus**" is my choice right now, it not only guides you through proper CPR compressions, but has a plastic lid that can be placed under the victim's shoulders which serves to keep the victim's head tilted back, keeping their airway open.*

Here's the four steps on how to use an AED:

1. Get the AED.
2. Open it.
3. Turn it on.
4. Listen to the voice prompts, follow instructions.

a. It will tell you to apply the adhesive patches to the person's chest, following the pictures on the patches for proper placement.
   b. It will tell you to *stay clear*, and not touch the person as it analyzes the heart rhythm.
   c. If a shock is needed it will charge up and then tell you to *stay clear* (don't touch the person) and push the flashing button to deliver the shock.

5. After the shock, you should then begin CPR. Every two minutes it will stop you and analyze the heart again, and perhaps shock them again. Just follow the voice prompts.

Some defibrillators, such as was mentioned on the previous page, will also guide the user in how to properly perform CPR!

*That's it. It's simple, and it is the only real hope this person has. You **must** have quick access to an AED, it **must** be used within the first few minutes of a cardiac arrest!*

•

<u>Note</u>: The defibrillator company(s) that get involved in this effort can discount the cost of their defibrillators due to the volume sold, and the cost will be insignificant to the final cost of the home and mortgage! The public service benefit and positive publicity for the homebuilders and for the defibrillator company(s) involved will be priceless!

~

First Aid

When it comes to *first aid*, most people don't know what to do. The AED is simple first aid to use in a cardiac arrest, but will you have one when you need it? *First aid* training will give you the knowledge to do the right thing even with limited or no equipment. In *Chapter Five* I mention a simple book on CPR that I wrote. That book also discusses the essential first aid information that everyone should know; I'll cover some of that here, in this little test:

First Aid Test:

Do you know what to do?

1. *You come home and find a loved one lying on the floor, you call out to them, they don't respond. They're lying face down. You roll them over and try to wake them up, they don't respond. What do you do now?*

   a. Call 9-1-1, wait for help to arrive.

   b. Call 9-1-1 then check to see if they are breathing and if they have a pulse, if they have a pulse but are not breathing, give them "rescue breathing" (one breath every 5 seconds.) If no breathing and no pulse, begin CPR. If you have an AED use that first!

2. An adult or child is choking on something. They have their hands to their throat, they can't speak, they are turning blue around their lips. What do you do now?

a. Call 9-1-1, wait for help to arrive.

b. Have someone call 9-1-1, slap them on the back hard, trying to get them to expel the object.

c. Move behind them, do the Heimlich maneuver.

d. Begin CPR.

3. *Your loved one seems confused, they are having trouble speaking, their words sound slurred. What do you do now?*

a. Call 9-1-1, wait for help to arrive.

b. Have them sit down. Don't lie them down. Call 9-1-1. Stay calm, try to keep them calm.

c. Give them some water, see if things improve. Maybe they are tired. Maybe it's a reaction to some medicine. Let them rest.

d. Call their doctor. Make an appointment, they should have a checkup.

I know, some of those choices seem silly, but many people will do c. or d. which could be fatal. We should always think the "worst case" when deciding what to do in a medical emergency, which usually means call 9-1-1. This could be a "stroke." A stroke is a brain problem, either a blood clot or a small ruptured vessel. This is life-threatening. High blood pressure is often a factor, lying them down could create more pressure in the brain and could make the stroke worse, keep them sitting up (choice b.) Rapid transport to the emergency room, or better yet, to a stroke center if available, is vital.

4. *You're alone watching TV, you begin to feel nauseated, you get sweaty, you have a little trouble catching your breath. What should you do?*

a. Call 9-1-1, wait for help to arrive.

b. Take some antacid if you have some. Relax.
Rest. This feeling is likely to go away soon.

c. Take this seriously, it could be the sign of a
heart attack.

d. Since you don't have chest pain, this isn't a
heart attack, so relax. Things like this usually go
away on their own.

e. Call 9-1-1, lie down, stay calm.

*This could be a trick question. You should have picked c. and e.
If we get proper medical help quickly we might prevent a heart
attack, or make sure it doesn't get worse. If we wait, we might
die. A heart attack does not always cause "pain." Laying down
may help to keep your heart and brain better oxygenated.*

5. **You've discovered someone who is on the floor
unresponsive (unconscious.) You aren't sure if
they are breathing, you think they may have just
taken a shallow breath, you aren't sure. You don't
know how to check a pulse properly, so you aren't
sure if they have a pulse or not. What should you
do?**

a. Call 9-1-1, wait for help to arrive, medical
professionals will need to figure this out.

b. Call 9-1-1 then begin CPR.

c.   Sit them up, keep shouting at them to "wake up."

d.   Place them on their side, to protect their airway in case they vomit.

Choice b. is correct. If we aren't <u>certain</u> that they are breathing adequately, and not certain they have a pulse, begin CPR. Never sit someone up who is unconscious, keep them lying down. "Recovery position" is the placement on their side, with their top leg bent to prop them up in that position, to help protect their airway if they vomit; recovery position is for someone unconscious who IS breathing and DOES have a pulse.

6.   Someone who is awake is struggling to breathe, they have noisy, wet sounding breathing, they are laying down. What do you do now?

a.   Call 9-1-1, wait for help to arrive.

b.   Sit them up, then call 9-1-1.

c.   Offer them a small drink of water, this might help clear their airway.

d.   Keep them lying down and call 9-1-1.

Choice b. is correct. People with trouble breathing should be kept sitting up. Don't give anyone having who is having trouble breathing or anyone who is not fully alert anything to drink.

7.   You have sat someone up who is having trouble breathing, and you have called 9-1-1. They

suddenly become unconscious. What do you do now?

    a.   Hold them up in a sitting position and wait for help to arrive.

    b.   Lay them down, check their pulse and breathing.

    c.   Place them in "recovery position."

We should lay them down, choice b. We would then check for breathing and pulse and do CPR if they are not breathing and have no pulse. If they are breathing, but have fainted, keep them lying down, and monitor their breathing and pulse, if their breathing or pulse stops, do CPR. Watch them, if they vomit, quickly put them on their side in 'recovery position.'

*How did you do? Some of this is not necessarily 'common sense' and you might not know what to do unless you were trained. These few questions cover some of the most important aspects of life-saving first aid. Knowing what to do keeps you from panicking. You'll be better able to think clearly and to do the right thing when you **know** you're doing the **right** thing. You should take a CPR and First Aid course, and/or read a book on these subjects. You need to be prepared, and you need to do the right thing, quickly and correctly in the event of a life-threatening emergency!*

*Notice that **none** of the answers were **ONLY** call 9-1-1, there were some important things to **do** that could make the difference between life and death.*

Chapter Four

A*LIVE* in Las Vegas!

Casinos and AED's

More than a decade ago *Las Vegas* began putting AED's in their casinos and training their security personnel how to use them.

Remember the dismal "save" rates by simply calling 9-1-1 for a cardiac arrest? FIVE PERCENT. In *Las Vegas* casinos they can get to a person who has collapsed in cardiac arrest and defibrillate them **within the first few minutes of their collapse**.

*What's the save rate for cardiac arrest in Las Vegas casinos? About **76%!***

This chapter is going to be short, because this part of the story is *simple*, we *know* what works. What they did in *Las Vegas* solved the survival problem that this book is all about. ***They simply got the AED to the victim in time***, in those first vital minutes. We can see the statistics in *Las Vegas*, they are clear, and *incredible*. That same story could be happening across our Nation, in our *homes*, as more and more new homes are equipped with AED's!

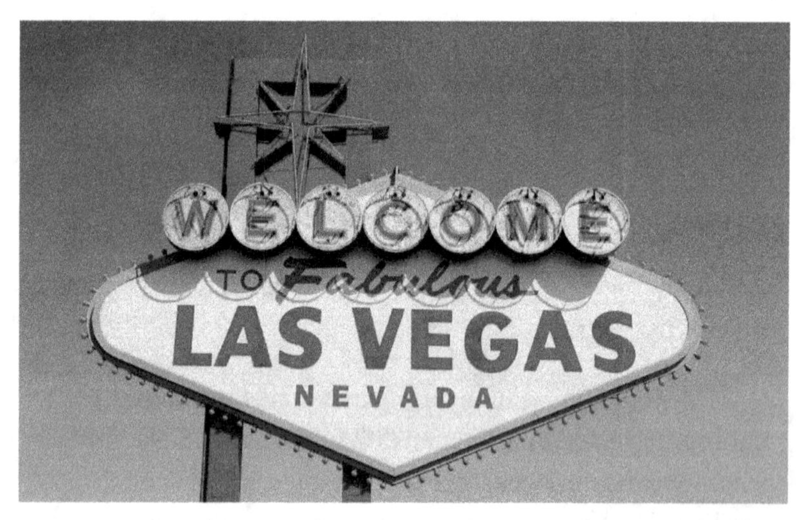

WELCOME
TO Fabulous
LAS VEGAS
NEVADA

Chapter Five

CPR *(Cardio-Pulmonary Resuscitation)*

Cardio = heart   Pulmonary = lungs

"Hand's Only" CPR is the simplest form of CPR. For adults, you put the heel of your hand on the middle of their chest, with the center of your palm in line with the nipple line, and you push down at least two inches deep, *which is harder than most people would think you should push*, and you push at a rate of about 100 times per minute, which is the beat of the *Bee Gees* song "Stayin Alive." That's it. No breaths, nothing else to think about, just push hard and fast and keep going.

~

My little book **"5-Minute CPR: A Paramedic's Guide to Simple CPR"** is inexpensive, is available at *Amazon,* and teaches Hands-Only CPR *and* basic First Aid in just 25 pages! It also makes a great, and life-saving, *gift* to all your friends and family!

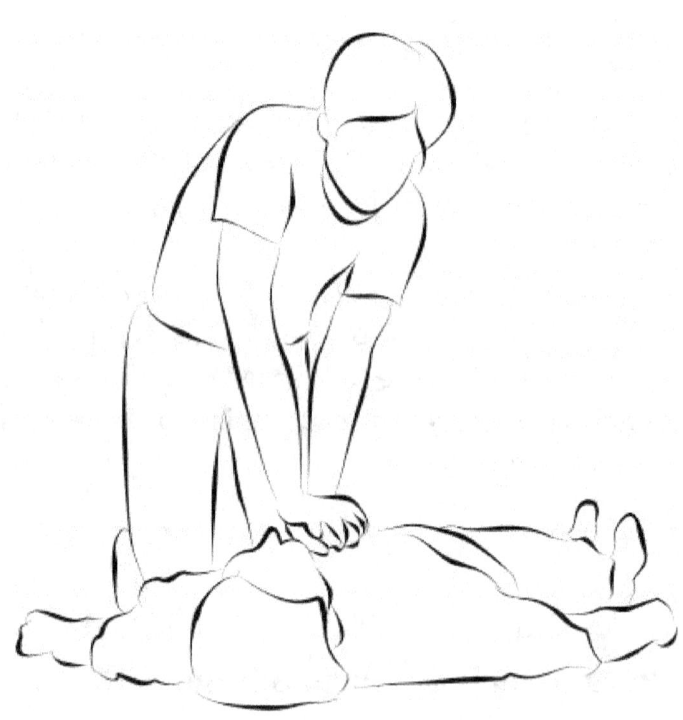

Chapter Six

The Pioneers of Life-Saving Home Building

On (date) (name of home builder) joined in this important effort and pledged to begin placing AED's in their new homes being built!

This was the beginning of a paradigm shift in saving lives from cardiac arrest…

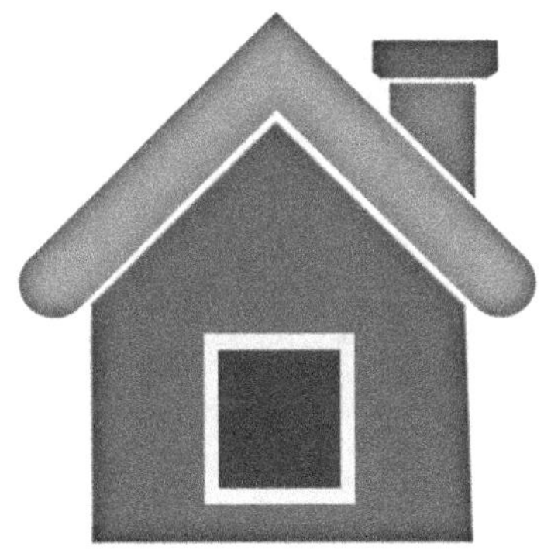

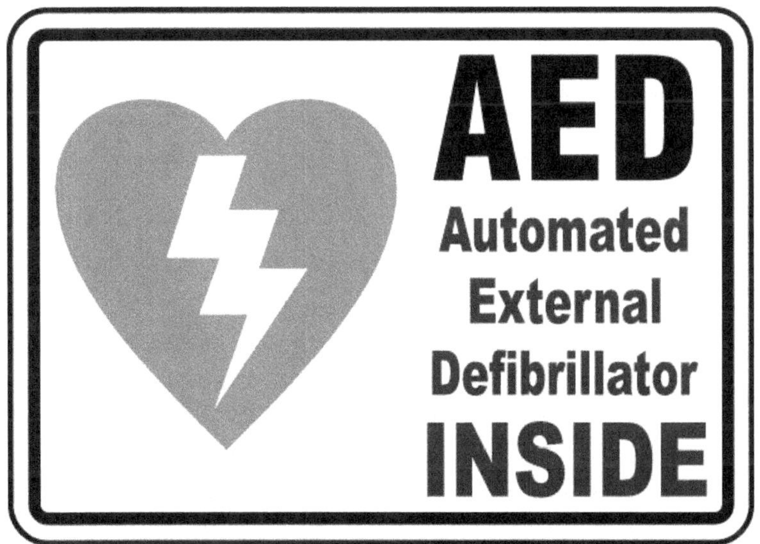

All it takes is a sticker on a door, and a defibrillator placed on a shelf in an existing cabinet in a new home; that's it.

A major defibrillator company (to be announced) should be excited to join this effort as we begin a new paradigm of Homebuilders as Lifesavers!

Our goal...

A movement begins; homebuilders become lifesavers as AEDs are placed in new homes being built.

About 350,000 people die each year from cardiac arrest.
*Nearly 80% of those cardiac arrests occur at **home**.* The *American Heart Association* estimates that raising our "save rates" from cardiac arrest from the current 5% to 20% would save ***50,000 to 100,000 lives every year!***

~

Will <u>you</u> be the first homebuilder to begin placing AEDs in their new homes?

Your company can spearhead this effort. Your company can take the lead to save lives in a way that only homebuilders can. Make your company THE homebuilder that started this lifesaving mission.

•

This is a BIG DEAL and I need your help.

If home builders would begin placing defibrillators (AEDs) in their new homes, we would begin an effort that would eventually save hundreds or thousands of lives.

<u>280,000 cardiac arrest deaths occur every year at HOME!</u>

The cost of adding an AED in a new home project is negligible.

*There is NO OTHER WAY to impact that figure of 280,000 dead **at home** each year from cardiac arrest; 9-1-1 services will arrive too late with their AED; the AED must be available and used **in the first three minutes** of a cardiac arrest for the best chance of survival!*

Please contact me so that we can discuss how *your company* can join this effort.

The positive publicity would be tremendous, and the impact on lives saved would be wonderful.

Lance Hodge, Paramedic • LanceHodge@outlook.com

Conclusion...

This book will be updated frequently, to reflect each of those homebuilders who join in this important effort.

I'll make certain the media know this is happening, I'll send a press release and a copy of this updated book to the major media outlets so that the public will recognize those companies who have recognized that *home building* can equal *life-saving*.

This simple change will be *profound*. Our future can be one in which a life-saving AED will be in *every* new home, and in this future many thousands of people will live that would otherwise have died. Other public and private efforts might follow, to get AED's in *existing* homes, and thousands more will live that would otherwise have died.

We will owe this brighter future to those innovative and far-sighted companies, those *homebuilders* who realized that being a successful corporation means more than just some bottom line, who realized something *amazing*, that *home building* could be more than the construction of some *house*, that it could represent the *meaning* of **home**; a place for families to live, and grow, and to thrive, and that the building of a *home* could also represent *saving lives*, and they boldly took the first steps toward this future.

Lance Hodge

The New England Journal of Medicine

Volume 343, Number 17, October 26, 2000

This study details survival rates in Las Vegas Casinos, and determines that defibrillation should occur in 3 minutes or less for the greatest chance of survival from cardiac arrest with ventricular fibrillation.

Survival in this limited study was 74% if defibrillation occurred in 3 minutes or less and dropped to 49% if defibrillation occurred after 3 minutes!

Note: 9-1-1 EMTs or Paramedics will almost *never* arrive in < 3 minutes!

YOU can be the <u>FIRST</u> homebuilder to join this life-saving movement and finally make a difference in how we save the lives of those who suffer a cardiac arrest:

The Pioneers of Life-Saving Home Building

On (date) (**YOUR COMPANY HERE**) began this important effort and pledged to begin placing AED's in their new homes being built!

This was the beginning of a paradigm shift in saving lives from cardiac arrest…

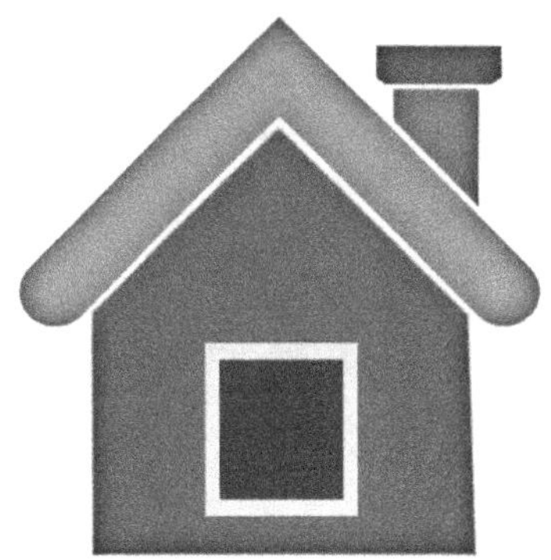

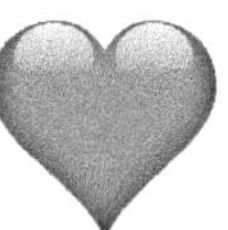

To those homebuilders, in advance, and to that brighter future; thank you!

Other books by Lance Hodge

5-Minute CPR:

A Paramedic's Guide to Simple CPR

~

Lost in the Woods: A Children's Survival Guide

~

A Paramedic's Guide: Wilderness First Aid

~

The Celebrity's Guide to Medical Security

~

A Kid's book on First Aid (1&2)

~

My BIG BOOK on First Aid and Safety (for kids)

Available at:

AMAZON.com, Booksamillion.com, Barnes & Noble, and other fine book sellers

Contact me:

LanceHodge@outlook.com